R POTTER

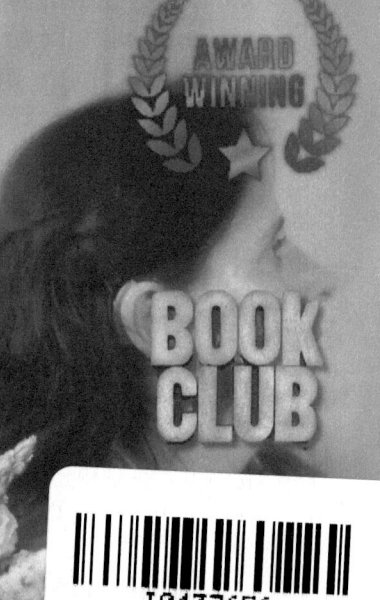

AWARD WINNING

BOOK CLUB

I0437656

ART OF LIVING

Skills for Navigating Life's Ups and Downs

978-1-4467-6393-3
Imprint: Lulu.com

9 781446 763933

For Steppie

THE ART OF LIVING: SKILLS FOR NAVIGATING LIFE'S UPS AND DOWNS"

W hen we think of the term 'resilience,' our minds often conjure images of a towering oak tree standing firm amidst a violent storm. Just as that tree stands unbowed despite the forces of nature, so too does the resilient individual weather life's myriad challenges. But how does one cultivate this resilience? How does one foster that inner strength which allows us to not just survive, but thrive in the face of adversity? This chapter seeks to answer those questions, guiding you toward understanding and embracing the concept of resilience in all its forms.

The True Meaning of Resilience

Resilience, at its core, isn't just about bouncing back from setbacks; it's about adapting and growing from them. It's the ability to endure, recover, and then evolve in response to adversity. Imagine water flowing down a mountain. When it encounters an obstacle, it finds a way around, over, or even through it. The water adapts, changes course, and continues on its journey, never halted for long by the barriers in its path.

Why Resilience Matters

The trials we face in life are inevitable, from personal struggles such as illness, loss, and financial hardships to global challenges like societal upheavals or natural disasters. Embracing resilience ensures that we can face these adversities head-on, armed with the knowledge that we possess the internal resources to overcome them.

Cultivating Your Inner Resilience

Self-awareness: Understand your emotions, triggers, and reactions. By recognizing how you react to stress and adversity, you can better prepare for and manage these situations.

Mindfulness and Meditation: Practices like mindfulness and meditation help keep us grounded, allowing us to approach challenges with a clear, calm mind.

Positive Relationships: Surround yourself with supportive friends and family. Having a strong support system provides a safety net during tough times.

Continuous Learning: Embrace a growth mindset. View challenges as opportunities to learn and grow, rather than insurmountable obstacles.

Physical Well-being: Regular exercise, a balanced diet, and adequate sleep are foundational to building resilience. A healthy body supports a healthy mind.

Setting Boundaries: Understand your limits and set boundaries. This protects your mental and emotional well-being.

Turning Challenges into Stepping Stones

Every challenge you face is an opportunity in disguise. It's a chance to learn more about yourself, to test your limits, and to grow stronger. By reframing adversity as a teacher rather than an enemy, you change the narrative of your life. You become the master of your destiny, using each stumbling block as a stepping stone to greater heights.

Conclusion

Life will always be filled with challenges. That's a given. But our response to those challenges is within our control. By embracing resilience, we equip ourselves with the tools to navigate life's ups and downs, ensuring that no matter what we face, we remain steadfast, adaptable, and ever-growing. As you journey through the subsequent chapters, keep the lessons of resilience close to your heart, for they will serve as

your compass in the tumultuous
seas of life.

In our quest to embrace life's adversities with resilience, one powerful ally stands out: the strength of positive thinking. Often, when we hear the term "positive thinking," our minds gravitate towards the clichéd notion of seeing the glass half full. However, this chapter goes beyond that surface-level understanding, diving deep into the realms of positive psychology and elucidating how a constructive mindset can truly reshape our lives.

What is Positive Psychology?

Positive psychology, a term coined by Dr. Martin Seligman, is a branch of psychology that studies the strengths and virtues that enable individuals and communities to thrive. Instead of focusing on deficits, disorders, and dysfunctions, positive psychology emphasizes strengths, solutions, and optimal functioning. It's not about denying the negatives in life but about focusing on and harnessing the positives.

The Cornerstones of Positive Thinking

Optimism: The belief that the future will be favorable and that good outcomes await, even in the face of adversity.

Gratitude: Recognizing and appreciating the good in life. This could be in the form of daily blessings, the kindness of others, or the beauty of nature.

Affirmation: Positive self-talk and constructive internal dialogues that reinforce self-worth and potential.

Visualization: Picturing favorable outcomes and

imagining the steps needed to achieve our goals.

How Positive Thinking Impacts Our Lives

Boosts Resilience: Positive thinkers recover from setbacks more quickly and are better equipped to deal with adversity.

Enhances Physical Health: Positive emotions and optimism are linked to a lower risk of chronic diseases, better immune function, and even a longer life.

Promotes Mental Well-being: Positive thinking is associated with lower levels of depression, increased life satisfaction, and greater overall well-being.

Improves Problem-Solving Abilities: A positive mindset

allows for more creative thinking and a broader range of possible solutions.

Cultivating a Positive Mindset

Challenge Negative Thoughts: Whenever you catch yourself thinking negatively, challenge those thoughts. Ask yourself if they're truly accurate, if they're the worst-case scenario, and what positive angles you haven't considered.

Practice Gratitude Daily: Keep a gratitude journal, noting down three things you're thankful for every day.

Surround Yourself with Positive Influences: Your environment plays a significant role in shaping your mindset.

Ensure that you're surrounded by positive influences and uplifting individuals.

Set Aside Time for Self-reflection: Regular introspection helps identify patterns in negative thinking and offers opportunities to address underlying issues.

Conclusion

The power of positive thinking isn't about ignoring life's challenges or masking pain with false positivity. It's about facing adversities with a hopeful heart and a mind that's open to solutions and growth. By cultivating a positive mindset, we set ourselves on a path where obstacles become opportunities, challenges become stepping stones, and life's ups and downs are met with grace, strength, and optimism. Remember, it's not what happens to us, but how we choose to respond, that truly defines our journey.

At a time when IQ tests and grades define a significant portion of our perceived intelligence, an equally, if not more important form of intelligence often gets overlooked: Emotional Intelligence (EI). This chapter takes you on a journey through the intricacies of EI, illustrating how it plays a crucial role in achieving success, not only professionally but, more importantly, in the realm of personal relationships and self-understanding.

What is Emotional Intelligence?

Emotional Intelligence, as coined by researchers Peter Salovey and John Mayer and later popularized by Daniel Goleman, refers to the ability to recognize, understand, manage, and regulate our emotions, as well as the emotions of others. It's about perceiving emotions correctly, using them appropriately, and managing both our own emotions and those of others effectively.

Components of Emotional Intelligence

Self-Awareness: Recognizing and understanding your own emotions as they arise. It's the cornerstone of EI because self-understanding paves the way for managing one's emotions.

Self-Regulation: Controlling and adapting your emotions, depending on the situation. This means not being overly reactive and thinking before acting.

Motivation: Being driven to fulfill your needs or achieve your goals, beyond money or recognition.

Empathy: Understanding and sharing the feelings of another. It's the ability to recognize emotions in others and to understand their perspective.

Social Skills: Building and managing healthy relationships, communicating clearly, and navigating social situations and conflicts.

Why Emotional Intelligence Matters

Personal Relationships: High EI leads to healthier and more fulfilling relationships as you can understand and cater to the emotional needs of your loved ones.

Professional Success: A person with high EI can navigate office politics, lead teams, and handle challenging situations effectively.

Mental Well-being: Recognizing and managing your emotions can lead to better mental health and lower levels of stress.

Decision Making: Emotions play a significant role in decision-making. Understanding them can lead to better and more informed choices.

Boosting Your Emotional Intelligence

Practice Active Listening: When someone speaks, listen with intent. This means not formulating your response while they're still talking, but genuinely trying to understand their perspective.

Keep a Feelings Journal: Documenting your emotions can help you understand patterns, triggers, and ways to manage them better.

Seek Feedback: Sometimes, we don't recognize our emotional reactions. Trusted friends or mentors can offer valuable insights.

Empathetic Engagement: Actively try to put yourself in someone else's shoes. It can be a loved one, a fictional character, or even a stranger.

Mindfulness and Meditation: These practices can

significantly increase your self-awareness and ability to regulate emotions.

Conclusion

In the ebb and flow of life, where relationships form the cornerstone of our experiences, Emotional Intelligence emerges as a beacon, guiding us through turbulent waters. It's not merely about being "book smart" or academically proficient; it's about understanding the human soul, starting with our own. By honing our Emotional Intelligence, we unlock doors to deeper connections, personal growth, and an enriched life, marked by understanding, empathy, and genuine success.

Mindfulness, a word that's become increasingly prevalent in our modern lexicon, traces its roots to ancient Buddhist practices. At its essence, it refers to a state of being present, fully engaged with the here and now. It means being attuned to our experience in the current moment, rather than being lost in thoughts about the past or anxieties about the future.

In our fast-paced world where multitasking has become the norm, our minds often juggle numerous tasks and thoughts simultaneously. This scatter-brained existence can lead to heightened stress, decreased efficiency, and a diminished ability to enjoy life's simple pleasures. Mindfulness offers an antidote to this, a bridge that connects us back to the richness of the present moment.

Imagine walking through a garden and being acutely aware

of the crunch of leaves underfoot, the scent of blooming flowers, the play of light and shadow through the trees, and the gentle caress of the wind. This heightened awareness, this deep connection with the present, is mindfulness in action.

The practice of mindfulness doesn't require a complete lifestyle overhaul. It's about making small, deliberate changes to our daily routines and habits. For starters, dedicating just a few minutes each day to focused breathing exercises can make a significant difference. During this time, the goal is to concentrate solely on one's breath, noticing the rhythm of inhalation and exhalation, and gently bringing the mind back whenever it wanders.

Another effective approach is the body scan meditation, where attention is gradually moved throughout the body, noting sensations, tensions, and relaxation. This practice not only enhances mindfulness but also helps in recognizing and releasing physical stress.

Mindfulness can also be woven into everyday activities. Whether it's savoring the flavors and textures of a meal, immersing oneself in the sensation of warm water during a shower, or truly listening when someone speaks, every moment offers an opportunity for mindful engagement.

The benefits of incorporating mindfulness into daily life are manifold. Research has shown that regular mindfulness practices can reduce symptoms in people suffering from anxiety, depression, and chronic pain. Mindfulness also strengthens the immune system, improves sleep quality, and heightens one's overall sense of well-being.

Beyond the physical and psychological advantages, mindfulness fosters a deep sense of gratitude and contentment. By anchoring ourselves in the present, we begin to notice and appreciate the multitude of blessings that often go unnoticed - from the beauty of a sunrise to the laughter of a loved one.

In conclusion, mindfulness is more than just a practice; it's a way of life. It's a conscious choice to engage fully with the present, to experience life in all its richness, and to navigate the world with a heightened sense of awareness, compassion, and gratitude. As we journey through the ups and downs of life, mindfulness serves as a grounding force, a gentle reminder to cherish the here and now.

In the tapestry of life, relationships are the threads that bind us together, providing a sense of belonging, support, and connection. They are the bedrock of our experiences, the mirrors that reflect back to us our joys, sorrows, strengths, and vulnerabilities. However, as with any intricate tapestry, these threads require care, attention, and understanding to maintain their strength and vibrancy.

Every relationship, whether with family, friends, or romantic partners, holds its unique set of challenges and rewards. At the foundation of every positive relationship is a shared understanding, mutual respect, open communication, and unwavering trust. And while these may sound like broad concepts, their application is seen in our everyday interactions.

Establishing healthy relationships begins with understanding oneself. Recognizing one's own needs, boundaries, strengths, and weaknesses enables clearer communication with others. When we understand what we seek from a relationship and what we can offer in return, the foundation becomes stronger and more transparent.

Open and honest communication is the lifeblood of any relationship. By expressing our feelings, needs, desires, and concerns openly, we allow for understanding and compromise. It's essential to remember that communication isn't just about speaking; it's equally about listening. Truly hearing what the other person has to say, without judgment or interruption, creates an environment of trust and mutual respect.

Trust, once established, becomes the cornerstone of any relationship. However, trust is fragile. It requires nurturing, consistency, and time. It's not just about being reliable but also about being vulnerable, about showing one's true self, warts and all. In the realm of romantic relationships, this vulnerability becomes even more profound. Sharing dreams, fears, joys, and sorrows paves the way for a deeper connection and understanding.

Yet, relationships aren't always smooth sailing. Disagreements and conflicts are natural and even healthy. They offer opportunities for growth, for understanding different viewpoints, and for strengthening the bond. It's not the absence of conflicts but the manner in which they are addressed and resolved that defines the health of a relationship. Empathy plays a crucial role here. Stepping into another's shoes, understanding their perspective, and finding common ground can turn disagreements into moments of shared growth.

Of course, relationships evolve over time. As individuals grow, change, and face different life stages, their relationships too undergo transformations. This evolution is natural and to be embraced. What remains constant, however, is the effort, understanding, and love that we pour into them.

In the journey of life, the relationships we build and nurture become our anchors, our sources of strength, and our reservoirs of joy. By investing time, patience, understanding, and love into them, we ensure that these threads in our life's tapestry remain strong, vibrant, and ever-lasting.

Navigating the diverse waters of human interaction demands a style of communication that's clear, respectful, and effective. At the heart of this style lies assertiveness–a balanced approach that stands midway between passive submission and aggressive confrontation. Assertive communication is about expressing oneself effectively and standing up for one's point of view, all while respecting the rights and beliefs of others.

Imagine a spectrum where on one end is passive communication, characterized by an inability or unwillingness to express oneself or stand up for one's rights. On the opposite end lies aggressive communication, which tends to violate the rights of others through dominating behaviors and words. Assertive communication beautifully balances these extremes, promoting an interaction style that's open, honest, and respectful.

The beauty of assertive communication lies in its emphasis on mutual respect. It's not just about getting one's point across but ensuring that the dialogue remains open and constructive. This becomes particularly important in situations of conflict or disagreement, where emotions might otherwise cloud judgment and hinder effective communication.

One of the first steps towards adopting an assertive communication style is self-awareness. Recognize your feelings and needs and take responsibility for them. Instead of saying, "You make me feel...," an assertive communicator might say, "I feel... when...". This approach acknowledges personal feelings and doesn't shift blame.

Another crucial aspect of assertive communication is clarity. Be specific about your needs or concerns. Instead of making vague statements, articulate precisely what you're feeling or what you need. This reduces the risk of misunderstandings and ensures that the message is clear.

Moreover, assertive communication often uses "I" statements. This not only promotes taking responsibility for one's feelings but also minimizes the chances of the listener becoming defensive. For instance, saying "I feel overwhelmed when I have too many tasks at once, and I would appreciate some assistance" is more effective and less confrontational than saying "You are giving me too much work."

But assertive communication isn't just about expressing one's own needs. It's equally about active listening. This means truly hearing what the other person has to say, not interrupting, and not jumping to conclusions. It's a two-way street, where both parties feel heard, valued, and respected.

In professional settings, assertive communication can help in clear articulation of ideas, effective teamwork, and conflict resolution. It sets the tone for a respectful work environment and can significantly impact career progression. In personal settings, it helps in establishing boundaries, ensuring mutual respect, and fostering deeper, more meaningful relationships.

In conclusion, assertive communication is a powerful tool in the arsenal of interpersonal skills. It helps bridge gaps, resolve conflicts, and establish meaningful connections. It's a skill that can be honed with practice, patience, and a genuine desire to engage in mutually respectful communication. In the dance of human interactions, assertiveness ensures that every voice is heard, every perspective valued, and every interaction is a step towards mutual understanding and respect.

Conflict, in its many forms, is an inescapable part of the human experience. Whether it arises from differing opinions, misunderstandings, or competing desires, conflict can strain relationships and create a sense of tension. However, when approached with the right mindset and tools, conflict can also provide opportunities for growth, deeper understanding, and improved communication.

Recognizing the inevitability of conflict is the first step towards handling it constructively. When we accept that disagreements are a natural part of relationships and can't always be avoided, we begin to see them as challenges to be solved rather than battles to be won. With this perspective, the focus shifts from assigning blame to seeking understanding.

One of the foundational techniques for resolving conflict

is active listening. This involves genuinely trying to understand the other person's perspective without immediately formulating a counter-argument. By giving the other person space to express themselves and showing that their feelings and opinions are valued, we can often defuse a situation before it escalates.

Equally important is the ability to communicate our own feelings and needs without resorting to accusations or negative language. This might mean using "I" statements to express how we feel, rather than making generalizations or pointing fingers. For example, saying "I feel hurt when you cancel our plans" is more conducive to a positive resolution than "You never prioritize our time together."

Taking a break can also be a valuable technique, especially when emotions run high. Sometimes, stepping away from a heated discussion for a short period can provide the clarity needed to approach the situation more constructively. It allows both parties to reflect, calm down, and come back with a renewed focus on resolving the conflict.

Another critical aspect of navigating conflict is seeking a compromise. This doesn't mean one party has to give up their stance entirely but finding a middle ground where both parties feel their needs are met. Compromise involves a willingness to adjust and an understanding that relationships often require give and take.

In situations where the conflict seems unresolvable, seeking external help can be beneficial. This could be in the form of a trusted friend or family member who can offer a fresh perspective or, in more severe cases, professional mediation or counseling.

Lastly, it's crucial to remember that every conflict, no matter how intense, provides a chance for growth. Every disagreement is an opportunity to understand our own reactions, biases, and triggers. It allows us to develop better communication skills, cultivate empathy, and deepen our connections with others.

In conclusion, navigating conflict is not about avoiding disagreements but about approaching them with an open heart and mind. It's about understanding that every relationship has its challenges, but with the right tools and mindset, these challenges can be turned into stepping stones for growth, deeper connection, and mutual understanding.

Money, often referred to as the "root of all evil," is paradoxically also one of the primary tools that facilitates our dreams, goals, and aspirations. Understanding and managing it well, therefore, is paramount not just for material success, but also for peace of mind and personal freedom. Let's delve into the fundamental principles of managing personal finances.

Understanding Your Financial Picture: Before one can chart a path forward, it's essential to understand where they stand. This means taking stock of all assets, liabilities, income sources, and expenditures. By obtaining a clear snapshot of your financial situation, you're better positioned to make informed decisions.

Budgeting: Once you know where your money is coming from and going to, you can start to exert more control over it. Creating a budget involves listing all your regular expenses, both fixed (like rent or mortgage) and variable (like entertainment or dining out), and matching them against your total income. The aim here is to ensure you're living within your means, ideally with a surplus that can be saved or invested.

Emergency Fund: Life is unpredictable. An unexpected medical expense, job loss, or major repair can set you back significantly if you're not prepared. Financial experts often recommend setting aside three to six months' worth of expenses in an easily accessible account to cover unforeseen events. This safety net can offer peace of mind and financial stability during turbulent times.

Saving: Beyond the emergency fund, saving regularly can help achieve larger goals, such as buying a house, traveling, or funding education. Setting clear goals and timeframes can make the saving process more structured and achievable.

Investing: While saving is about preserving capital, investing is about growing it. The world of investment offers various opportunities, from stocks and bonds to real estate and mutual funds. Each comes with its own risk-reward profile. As a general rule, investments that offer higher returns also come with higher risks. Starting early and being consistent can harness the power of compound interest, making money work harder for you over time.

Minimizing Debt: While certain debts, like student loans or mortgages, can be considered "good" debts because they represent an investment in the future, high-interest debts, especially from credit cards, can be financially draining. Prioritizing paying off high-interest debts and avoiding unnecessary borrowing can lead to a healthier financial future.

Staying Informed: The financial landscape is always evolving. From tax law changes to new investment opportunities, staying updated is crucial for making informed decisions. This doesn't mean one needs to become a finance expert, but regularly reading reputable finance news sources or consulting with a financial advisor can be beneficial.

Review and Adjust: As with all things in life, personal finance requires periodic review. Changes in income, lifestyle, family size, or goals can necessitate adjustments to the budget, savings, or investments.

In conclusion, personal finance management is a journey, not a destination. Regardless of one's financial situation, age, or goals, the principles outlined above can provide a roadmap for navigating the intricacies of money management. When harnessed effectively, money becomes more than just currency—it becomes a tool for realizing dreams, ensuring security, and fostering personal growth.

In the hustle and bustle of modern life, the pursuit of well-being often leans heavily towards physical health, inadvertently overshadowing its equally crucial counterpart:

mental health. Our mental state, intertwined with our emotions, thoughts, and perceptions, significantly impacts our overall quality of life. Prioritizing self-care is an act of honoring and nurturing this delicate balance of our psyche.

Understanding Mental Health: At its core, mental health is about emotional, psychological, and social well-being. It dictates how we think, feel, and act. It also helps determine how we handle stress, relate to others, and make choices. Just as one might suffer from a cold or a physical injury, mental health can fluctuate, and disturbances like depression, anxiety, or stress disorders can arise.

Breaking the Stigma: Recognizing the importance of mental health means dismantling societal stigmas surrounding it. Accepting and understanding that mental health challenges are as real and valid as physical ailments is the first step towards fostering a supportive environment for oneself and others.

Signs and Signals: Paying attention to sudden or prolonged changes in one's thoughts, emotions, or behaviors can be indicative of underlying mental health issues. Whether it's prolonged sadness, excessive worry, changes in sleeping or eating patterns, or social withdrawal, acknowledging these signs is crucial.

Self-Care Rituals: Incorporating regular self-care practices can act as preventive measures, bolstering mental resilience. This might include activities like meditation, journaling, engaging in hobbies, or simply taking time off to relax and rejuvenate.

Setting Boundaries: In an interconnected world, setting clear personal and professional boundaries can protect one's mental space. This might mean logging off from social media, saying 'no' when overwhelmed, or designating specific times for relaxation.

Seeking Professional Help: There's immense strength in recognizing when help is needed. Therapists, counselors, and psychiatrists offer professional support, providing coping mechanisms and therapeutic strategies to navigate mental health challenges.

Community and Connection: Engaging with supportive communities, whether they are friends, family, or support groups, can offer solace and understanding. Sharing experiences, feelings, or simply being there for one another can significantly alleviate mental burdens.

Physical Health and Mental Well-being: The connection between physical health and mental well-being is profound. Regular exercise, a balanced diet, adequate sleep, and avoiding alcohol, drugs, and other substances can significantly impact one's mental state, offering clarity, energy, and resilience.

Mindfulness and Grounding Practices: Activities like yoga, deep breathing exercises, or mindfulness meditation can anchor the mind, providing a calming refuge from the chaos of everyday life.

Educate and Advocate: Being informed about mental health, its challenges, and ways to support oneself and others can foster empathy and understanding in wider society. Advocating for mental health awareness can shift societal perceptions and bring about tangible change.

In conclusion, mental health, often dubbed the "silent pillar" of well-being, holds immense sway over our life's quality. Prioritizing self-care and mental well-being is not a luxury but a necessity. In nurturing our minds, we pave the way for richer, fuller, and more harmonious lives, where challenges are faced with resilience, joy is embraced with open arms, and every moment holds the promise of growth and discovery.

The ancient Romans coined the phrase "Mens sana in corpore sano," which translates to "A sound mind in a sound body." This timeless wisdom underscores the inextricable link between physical health and mental and emotional well-being. Cultivating physical health isn't just about appearance or athleticism–it's a holistic approach to ensuring the body operates at its optimal level, creating a foundation for every other aspect of life.

The Pillars of Physical Health: Physical health can broadly be divided into several areas: muscular strength and endurance, cardiovascular endurance, flexibility, nutrition, and sleep. Each component plays a vital role in overall well-being and requires individual attention.

Exercise as a Keystone: Regular physical activity has multifaceted benefits–it boosts mood, improves cardiovascular health, strengthens muscles, enhances flexibility, and aids in weight management. It's not about adopting the latest fitness trend but finding a consistent routine that you enjoy, whether it's walking, swimming, dancing, or weight training.

Nutrition: Fuel for the Body: What we eat significantly impacts our energy levels, immune system function, mood, and overall health. Consuming a balanced diet rich in whole foods, like vegetables, fruits, lean proteins, and whole grains, ensures the body receives essential nutrients. Hydration, often overlooked, plays a pivotal role in bodily functions from digestion to cognitive performance.

Sleep: The Restoration Period: Often sacrificed in the hustle of modern life, sleep is when the body repairs, restores, and rejuvenates. Achieving 7-9 hours of quality sleep for adults is crucial for cognitive function, emotional regulation, and physical health.

Posture and Ergonomics: In an age dominated by screens and desk jobs, understanding and practicing proper posture can prevent a myriad of musculoskeletal problems. Ergonomic workspaces and regular breaks can mitigate issues stemming from prolonged sitting or repetitive motions.

The Power of Rest: Active rest days, where one might engage in light activities or stretching, can aid recovery and prevent burnout. Listening to one's body and understanding when to push and when to rest is integral to long-term physical health.

Prevention and Regular Check-ups: Routine medical check-ups, screenings, and being proactive about health can detect potential issues before they become significant problems. Regular dental checks, eye exams, and age-appropriate screenings ensure that you're not just reacting to health issues but preemptively addressing them.

Holistic Approaches: Complementary therapies such as massage, acupuncture, or chiropractic care can offer additional avenues to physical well-being. While they shouldn't replace traditional medical care, they can be integrated into a holistic health regimen.

The Mind-Body Connection: Physical activities like Tai Chi, Yoga, or Pilates emphasize the harmony between mind and body, offering both physical benefits and mental relaxation.

Adapting and Evolving: As life progresses, our physical needs and abilities change. Adapting to these changes, whether it's switching exercise routines, modifying diets, or addressing age-related health concerns, ensures continuous well-being.

In conclusion, cultivating physical well-being is a lifelong journey that requires attention, consistency, and adaptability. A robust physical foundation not only ensures longevity but greatly enhances the quality of life, allowing us to engage with the world with vitality, enthusiasm, and joy.

We are inherently social beings. From the dawn of civilization, humans have thrived in communities, relying on one another for sustenance, protection, and companionship. This intrinsic need for connection has evolved over the millennia but remains as vital as ever. Our community shapes our worldview, offers support during challenging times, and provides moments of joy and celebration in life's highs.

The word 'community' extends beyond geographical boundaries or familial ties. It encompasses groups we choose and those we're born into. From professional networks, religious congregations, hobby clubs, to close-knit neighborhoods, every community serves a distinct purpose in our lives.

Modern life, with its digital interconnectedness, offers unprecedented opportunities to form and nurture communities. Social media platforms, online forums, and virtual meetups have blurred physical distances, enabling individuals to find their tribe regardless of location. While these digital connections are invaluable, they are most enriching when complemented by tangible, real-world interactions.

Community and connection's benefits are vast. Being part of a community offers a sense of belonging, reducing feelings of isolation or loneliness. These social networks act as a safety net, offering emotional, and sometimes even financial or physical support. Sharing experiences, knowledge, or resources within a community fosters personal growth and collective well-being. Moreover, connections often bring about a shared purpose or goal, providing direction and meaning to individual lives.

However, it's essential to choose and nurture communities that align with our values and aspirations. Not all groups or connections are beneficial. Some might foster negativity, prejudice, or pull us away from our true selves. Being discerning in our affiliations and ensuring mutual respect and growth is crucial for personal well-being.

Furthermore, as valuable as it is to be a part of various communities, it's equally crucial to contribute actively. Communities thrive on reciprocity. Offering our skills, time, or simply a listening ear enriches the collective and enhances our sense of purpose and belonging.

In essence, community and connection are the tapestries that enrich the fabric of our lives. They root us, uplift us, challenge us, and celebrate us. As the African proverb goes, "If you want to go fast, go alone. If you want to go far, go together." In the journey of life, our communities and connections ensure we go both far and deep, enriching every step along the way.

L ife, with all its beauty and wonder, is also inherently unpredictable. Change is the only true constant. Whether it's a job loss, moving to a new city, health challenges, or even smaller everyday adjustments, we all face change and uncertainty. How we respond to these shifts can define our experiences and influence our overall well-being.

Change can often be unsettling. Even positive changes, like a promotion or the birth of a child, come with their set of challenges. Human beings are creatures of habit, and deviations from the known can induce anxiety and stress. However, it's this very unpredictability that adds depth, learning, and growth to our lives.

Adapting to change requires a mix of resilience, flexibility, and a positive mindset. When confronted with unforeseen circumstances, it's beneficial to approach them not as insurmountable obstacles but as opportunities for growth. Every challenge comes with its set of lessons, and by embracing them, we often discover strengths and facets of ourselves we were previously unaware of.

It's also essential to acknowledge and accept the emotions that come with change. Denying feelings of fear, sadness, or anxiety can be counterproductive. Instead, allowing ourselves to feel, process, and then channel these emotions constructively can be therapeutic. Talking to someone, whether it's a trusted friend or a professional, can provide clarity and perspective.

Another crucial aspect of navigating change is to maintain a certain level of routine or consistency. While it's vital to be flexible, having some constants in daily life can provide a sense of stability and normalcy amidst the chaos.

Lastly, focusing on the present can significantly alleviate the anxiety of uncertainty. While it's essential to plan and be prepared, incessant worrying about future outcomes, especially those beyond our control, can be draining. Mindfulness practices, like meditation or deep breathing exercises, can be invaluable in grounding oneself in the present moment.

In retrospect, many find that the periods of most profound change and uncertainty in their lives also coincide with significant growth, self-discovery, and even unforeseen opportunities. Embracing change, with all its challenges and opportunities, is an integral aspect of the art of living. It reminds us of the transient nature of existence and the endless possibilities that every moment holds.

In the voyage of life, the quest for knowledge is both an anchor and a compass. From the cradle to the grave, the potential for learning never ceases. Lifelong learning isn't merely about academic pursuits; it's a mindset, a commitment to personal evolution and self-improvement.

From a very young age, formal education shapes our foundation, imparting essential knowledge and skills. But the real education, the one that shapes character and broadens horizons, often happens outside classroom walls. Every interaction, experience, and even setback provides a rich tapestry of lessons.

The modern era, often referred to as the information age, offers unparalleled opportunities for continuous learning. Digital platforms, online courses, podcasts, and webinars have democratized education, making it accessible to anyone with an internet connection. But learning isn't restricted to these platforms. Simple daily habits, like reading, engaging in stimulating conversations, or even trying out a new hobby, contribute to personal growth.

Lifelong learning enriches the mind and the soul. It fosters adaptability, a crucial trait in a rapidly evolving world. By staying curious and open to new knowledge, one remains relevant in professional spheres and keeps the mind agile and young. This continuous quest for knowledge also enhances self-awareness and broadens perspectives, facilitating a deeper understanding of oneself and the world.

But more than the practical benefits, learning feeds the innate human curiosity. It adds depth to existence, turning the mundane into wonder. Whether it's understanding the cosmos's vastness, a new culture's intricacies, or the workings of the human mind, learning illuminates and enriches our journey on this planet.

To commit to lifelong learning is to commit to a life of wonder, challenge, and growth. It's to recognize that the horizon of knowledge is infinite, and every step towards it, no matter how small, is a step towards a more fulfilled existence.

Letting go is an integral aspect of human experience, often intertwined with the most profound moments of our lives. It encompasses a range of emotions and actions: from releasing past traumas and forgiving oneself and others, to accepting the impermanence of life and gracefully moving past losses or setbacks.

At its core, the act of letting go is a process of liberation. By holding onto past regrets, resentments, or even idealized memories, we encase ourselves in a prison of our own making. These chains, often invisible, can hinder personal growth, wellbeing, and the ability to fully engage with the present.

However, the act of letting go isn't about negating or undermining the significance of past experiences or feelings. It's about acknowledging them, understanding their impact, and then choosing to release the weight they might carry. This release, while it sounds simple on paper, can be one of the most challenging yet rewarding endeavors one undertakes.

One of the first steps towards letting go is self-awareness. Understanding what and why we hold onto certain feelings or memories can provide clarity. Sometimes, it's fear of the future or an idealized version of the past that makes us cling. At other times, it could be unresolved emotions or traumas.

Acceptance follows awareness. Accepting that certain things are beyond our control, that life is inherently unpredictable, and that every experience, good or bad, contributes to the tapestry of our being, can be therapeutic. It creates a grounding from which the act of releasing becomes possible.

Letting go also extends to material possessions. In a consumer-driven world, it's easy to attach our worth or happiness to things. Periodically evaluating what truly adds value to our lives and letting go of excess can lead to a more focused and harmonious existence.

The beauty of letting go is in the space it creates - space for new experiences, relationships, and personal growth. It's a reaffirmation of the impermanence of life and a testament to human resilience and adaptability. Through the act of releasing, we often find deeper connections to ourselves, others, and the world around us, embodying the essence of the art of living.

In the hustle and bustle of modern life, moments of solitude have become increasingly rare. Yet, these moments, when we step away from external stimuli and immerse ourselves in introspection, hold profound value. Solitude isn't about isolation or loneliness. It's a conscious choice to spend time with oneself, to dive deep into the depths of one's mind, emotions, and aspirations.

For many, the idea of solitude can be daunting. The silence and lack of distraction, rather than offering peace, can amplify inner tumult. But it's precisely this confrontation with oneself, the addressing of innermost thoughts and feelings, that makes solitude so transformative.

Regular periods of solitude and reflection can offer clarity. In the absence of external influences, we often find authentic answers to pressing questions, solutions to problems that seemed insurmountable, or even profound realizations about our desires and goals. Solitude offers a mirror, reflecting the most genuine version of ourselves.

Beyond problem-solving, these moments also foster creativity. Many great thinkers, artists, and innovators have attested to the power of solitude in birthing new ideas and perspectives. The mind, when given space, can wander, explore, and create in unexpected and beautiful ways.

Solitude also strengthens emotional resilience. By spending time alone, we learn to find contentment within, reducing our dependency on external validations or stimuli for happiness. This intrinsic sense of worth and contentment can be a beacon during challenging times.

However, embracing solitude requires intention. It's easy to fill every waking moment with tasks, entertainment, or social interactions, especially in a digitally connected world. Setting aside dedicated periods for reflection, whether through meditation, nature walks, journaling, or simply sitting in silence, can be profoundly enriching.

In essence, solitude is a celebration of one's company. It's a realization that while connections and experiences shape our journey, the relationship with oneself is the foundation. By nurturing this relationship, by valuing moments of solitude and reflection, we not only enhance our understanding of ourselves but also deepen our connections with the world around us.

G ratitude is a deceptively simple emotion, often overshadowed by more intense feelings of joy, sorrow, anger, or desire. Yet, it is one of the most potent forces that can shape our outlook on life, health, and relationships. At its core, gratitude is about recognizing and appreciating the value in both big and small moments, the kindness of others, and even the challenges that lead to growth.

In a world that constantly pushes us to desire more, to climb higher, and to compare ourselves to others, it's easy to lose sight of what we already possess. This constant striving, while commendable in its ambition, can also lead to feelings of inadequacy or a sense that we're perpetually lacking. Gratitude offers a counter-narrative, suggesting that perhaps, in many ways, we have enough.

Embracing a gratitude-centric approach doesn't mean being complacent or ignoring genuine problems. Instead, it's about shifting our focus. By consciously recognizing and appreciating positive elements in our lives, we can balance our natural tendency to dwell on the negative. Over time, this can lead to a more optimistic outlook, improved mental well-being, and a heightened sense of life satisfaction.

Simple practices can cultivate a sense of gratitude. Maintaining a gratitude journal, where one notes down things they're thankful for daily, can be transformative. Expressing appreciation to loved ones, or even strangers, not only fosters positive relationships but also reinforces feelings of gratitude within.

Scientific studies have started to unveil the benefits of gratitude. People who regularly practice gratitude have been found to have lower stress levels, better immune function, and even improved sleep. These benefits, while secondary, underscore the profound impact of this simple emotion.

Furthermore, gratitude has the power to strengthen communities. When people feel appreciated and recognized, they're more likely to engage positively, fostering a sense of belonging and mutual respect.

In the grand tapestry of life, with its ups and downs, joys and sorrows, gratitude serves as a gentle reminder of the beauty that exists, often in the most unexpected places. It whispers to us that while there's always more to achieve or desire, there's also so much to cherish right now. And in this recognition lies a profound sense of peace and fulfillment.

L ife is a delicate dance of relationships. From family and friends to coworkers and acquaintances, our interactions form the rhythm of our days. While these connections enrich our lives, adding layers of joy, support, and understanding, they also come with challenges. One of the most vital, yet often overlooked, aspects of healthy relationships is the setting and respecting of boundaries.

Boundaries are the invisible lines that define our personal space, both physically and emotionally. They represent our values, limits, and self-worth. When these boundaries are recognized and respected, they foster a sense of security and mutual respect in relationships. Conversely, when they're crossed or ignored, they can lead to feelings of discomfort, resentment, or even violation.

Understanding and setting personal boundaries begins with self-awareness. Each individual's boundaries might differ based on their experiences, values, and personal comfort levels. What feels intrusive to one person might be perfectly acceptable to another. It's essential to reflect on and understand where one draws the line, be it in terms of personal space, time, emotional energy, or even topics of conversation.

Once these boundaries are understood, the next step is communication. Clearly conveying your boundaries is essential. It's neither confrontational nor selfish. Instead, it's an act of self-respect and a signal to others about how you wish to be treated. Just as we expect others to respect our boundaries, it's equally important to recognize and respect theirs.

In certain situations, particularly in close relationships or positions of power dynamics, boundary violations can be subtle or even unintentional. Here, open dialogue becomes crucial. Expressing feelings without assigning blame, using "I" statements, and seeking understanding can help navigate these nuanced situations.

Maintaining boundaries also extends to our digital lives. In an era of constant connectivity, it's easy to feel overwhelmed or overexposed. Setting limits on digital communication, curating one's online presence, and respecting the digital boundaries of others are modern-day essentials.

Boundaries, at their core, are an affirmation of self-worth. They signal that one values themselves enough to protect their well-being. They're also a testament to the value one places on their relationships, as mutual respect and understanding are cornerstones of any healthy connection. By balancing the needs of self and others, boundaries allow for deeper, more fulfilling relationships, enriching the dance of life.

Change is the only constant in life. From the shifts in personal circumstances to the broader changes in society and the environment, adaptability becomes a key trait to navigate the ever-evolving landscape of our existence. Being adaptable doesn't mean losing one's essence or compromising on values. It's the ability to adjust to new conditions while staying anchored in core beliefs.

Adaptability is often seen as the domain of the young, with age stereotypically bringing rigidity. Yet, the capacity to adapt isn't bound by age but by mindset. Those who retain a curious, open-minded approach to life tend to navigate changes with greater ease, irrespective of how many years they've lived.

Several elements contribute to adaptability. First and foremost is the acceptance of change. Resisting or denying change often leads to stress and frustration. By acknowledging the inevitability of change, one can approach it not as an adversary but as a part of life's natural flow.

Flexibility in thinking and action is another facet of adaptability. This involves looking at situations from multiple perspectives, being open to new information, and being willing to adjust one's approach based on the current context. It's about recognizing that there isn't always a singular 'right' way, but multiple paths that can lead to a desired outcome.

Cultivating a growth mindset, where challenges are seen as opportunities for growth rather than insurmountable obstacles, also fosters adaptability. It fuels the drive to learn, evolve, and rise to new occasions, turning setbacks into setups for future successes.

While adaptability aids in navigating external changes, it's also a tool for personal growth. Each adaptation, each adjustment made in the face of change, adds a layer to one's character, enriching the personal narrative.

The beauty of adaptability lies in its duality. It's both a shield and a compass. As a shield, it protects from the potential negative impacts of unexpected changes, allowing one to stay resilient. As a compass, it guides through unfamiliar terrains, opening up new horizons and experiences.

In the grand journey of life, filled with its twists and turns, adaptability is the wind beneath the wings, allowing us to soar even when the skies seem uncertain. It embodies the essence of the art of living, turning life's unpredictability from a challenge into an adventure.

Amidst the vast universe, on a small blue planet, our individual lives may sometimes seem insignificant. Yet, each day is a unique tapestry of experiences, emotions, and interactions, all woven together by a singular thread: purpose. While grand ambitions and life-changing moments often take the limelight, there is profound meaning to be found in the everyday, in the seemingly mundane.

Purpose isn't just about the major milestones or the monumental decisions. It's also about the small choices we make daily, the habits we cultivate, the kindness we extend, and the passions we pursue, even if only for a few minutes each day. It's about finding joy and significance in the ordinary, recognizing that each moment, no matter how routine, adds to the richness of life.

Every morning, when the alarm rings, is an opportunity to infuse purpose into the day. It might be through a morning ritual, be it meditation, reading, or simply sipping a cup of tea while watching the sunrise. These rituals ground us, offering a moment of reflection and intention before the day unfolds.

The conversations we have, even the briefest of exchanges, can be imbued with purpose. By being present, truly listening, and engaging with empathy, we can transform ordinary interactions into meaningful connections. The tasks we undertake, from cooking a meal to tending to a garden or even organizing a workspace, can become acts of love, creativity, or service when done with intention.

Finding purpose in the everyday is also about gratitude, about recognizing and appreciating the myriad of blessings that often go unnoticed. The warmth of the sun, the aroma of a freshly cooked meal, the laughter of a loved one - all these are daily miracles that add depth and joy to our existence.

For those feeling adrift, seeking a grand purpose or calling, it might be beneficial to shift the gaze from the horizon to the immediate surroundings. Often, the purpose we seek is not in some distant future or lofty goal, but right here, in the present moment, waiting to be acknowledged.

In the end, life's beauty isn't just in its peak moments but also in its valleys and plateaus. By finding purpose in the everyday, we not only enrich our own lives but also touch the lives of those around us, turning the ordinary into the extraordinary.

Creativity is often misunderstood as a gift reserved for artists, writers, or musicians. In reality, it's an inherent quality within each of us, waiting to be expressed in myriad ways. It's not just about creating art or literature; it's about viewing the world through a lens of possibility, innovation, and originality.

While certain professions demand obvious creative outputs, every individual, regardless of their job or daily routine, can integrate creativity into their life. It's about breaking free from monotony, exploring new avenues, and approaching problems with a fresh perspective.

Daily routines, while providing structure, can sometimes become stifling. Introducing small changes can spark creativity. It could be as simple as taking a different route to work, rearranging furniture, or trying out a new recipe. These shifts, though minor, can provide a fresh perspective and break the cycle of repetitiveness.

Challenging oneself is another avenue to foster creativity. Stepping outside of one's comfort zone, be it by learning a new skill, taking up a hobby, or even engaging in debates on unfamiliar topics, can stimulate the mind and unlock new ideas.

Diverse experiences feed creativity. Engaging with different cultures, reading varied genres of books, or even listening to different styles of music can introduce new concepts and viewpoints. This eclectic mix of experiences enriches the mind, offering a vast canvas for creative expression.

It's also essential to provide space for creativity to flourish. This means setting aside time for reflection, daydreaming, and even boredom. In an age of constant stimulation, moments of stillness become the crucible for creative thoughts.

Collaboration is another potent tool for nurturing creativity. Bouncing ideas off others, working on group projects, or simply discussing dreams and aspirations can lead to the merging of different perspectives, resulting in unique and innovative solutions.

Lastly, it's crucial to understand that creativity is a process, not an end result. It's about the journey, the exploration, and the joy of discovery. Mistakes, failures, and detours are all part of this journey. Instead of being disheartened by them, embracing them as stepping stones can lead to unexpected and beautiful destinations.

By weaving creativity into the fabric of daily life, one doesn't just add color and zest to their days but also paves the way for innovation, problem-solving, and a deeper connection with the world around them.

Time is the most precious and finite resource we have. Yet, in the modern hustle, the value of time often gets overshadowed by the illusion of busyness. Racing against the clock, we forget to savor the moments, to live them fully. This chapter delves into the art of making every moment count, ensuring that the legacy of time we leave behind is rich with meaning and experiences.

Understanding the value of time starts with introspection. What are the moments that you cherish the most? Often, they are not the ones filled with grand achievements but the ones filled with love, laughter, and genuine connection. It's the unexpected conversations, the serene walks, the joy of a shared meal, or the tranquility of a silent night.

Prioritizing quality over quantity is essential. Spending hours at a task doesn't necessarily make it valuable. Sometimes, a few moments of undivided attention can be more impactful than hours of distracted effort. Whether it's in relationships, work, or personal pursuits, depth often holds more value than breadth.

Mindfulness plays a pivotal role in making moments count. Being fully present, savoring each sensation, emotion, and thought allows one to truly live in the moment. It transforms mundane routines into memorable experiences, ensuring that no moment goes by unnoticed or unappreciated.

Delegation and prioritization are crucial skills in the efficient use of time. Not every task deserves your energy. By focusing on what truly matters and delegating or letting go of the rest, you can ensure that your time is spent on activities that align with your values and aspirations.

Embracing spontaneity adds a zest to life. While planning is essential, sometimes the most memorable moments arise from unplanned adventures, from saying 'yes' to the unexpected. These moments, filled with surprise and wonder, add a unique flavor to the tapestry of time.

Lastly, the legacy of time is not just about the moments we live but also the moments we give. Acts of kindness, of service, of love, leave an indelible mark on the sands of time. They transform fleeting moments into lasting memories, ensuring that the legacy we leave behind is one of meaning, connection, and joy.

In the grand theater of life, time is both the script and the director. How we choose to spend it, how we make every moment count, determines the story we weave and the legacy we leave behind.

Mortality is an inevitable aspect of the human condition, yet it remains one of the most challenging topics to confront. It serves as a profound reminder of the transience of our existence, prompting questions about the meaning of life, the nature of legacy, and the intricacies of grief. Embracing the journey's end isn't about dwelling on the melancholic notion of an ending, but rather acknowledging it as a fundamental part of life, lending urgency and significance to our days.

Accepting mortality begins with recognizing its inevitability. Every life, no matter how grand or humble, shares this common endpoint. Rather than viewing it with fear, embracing it can provide a unique clarity, a perspective that magnifies the importance of each moment and the value of authentic connections.

Conversations about mortality, though often avoided, can be deeply healing and illuminating. They provide an opportunity for reflection, for expressing wishes, for sharing fears, and for finding comfort in shared experiences. By bringing these conversations into the open, we can demystify death and approach it with a sense of understanding and preparedness.

Legacy is often intertwined with our perceptions of mortality. How do we want to be remembered? What impact do we wish to leave behind? Reflecting on these questions allows us to lead a life aligned with our deepest values, ensuring that our influence extends beyond our time.

Grief, as a response to the impermanence of life, is both complex and deeply personal. It's a testament to the depth of connections, to the love and bonds shared. By allowing oneself to grieve, to feel the full spectrum of emotions, we honor the memories and the significance of lost connections.

Yet, amidst the contemplation of mortality, there's an invitation to celebrate life. To cherish its highs and lows, its joys and sorrows, its love and heartbreak. By accepting the journey's end, we're prompted to live the journey itself with greater intention, passion, and authenticity.

In the grand narrative of existence, mortality adds

poignancy, reminding us of the fleeting nature of moments, urging us to live them with utmost sincerity. By embracing the journey's end, we don't succumb to despair but rise with a renewed vigor to make every chapter of our story meaningful and profound.

As the sun sets on the horizon of our narrative, we find ourselves at a pivotal juncture, looking back at the vast landscape of experiences, emotions, and memories that have shaped our journey. The Art of Living, as intricate and multifaceted as it is, finds its true essence not just in the moments lived but also in the wisdom drawn from those moments.

Each life is a unique blend of joys and sorrows, triumphs and challenges, hopes and heartbreaks. Yet, amid the diversity of experiences, there emerges a universal thread - the quest for understanding, for meaning, for connection. It's in this quest that we often find the most profound lessons, insights that illuminate the path ahead.

Reflection, as an act, is both an anchor and a compass. It roots us in our experiences, allowing us to savor memories, to mourn losses, and to cherish victories. At the same time, it guides our future, helping us make informed choices, avoid past pitfalls, and pursue paths that align with our deepest aspirations.

Drawing wisdom from life's experiences isn't about harboring regrets or getting trapped in the past. Instead, it's about recognizing patterns, celebrating growth, and acknowledging areas of improvement. It's about taking stock of where we've been, where we are, and where we wish to go.

Moreover, the tapestry of reflection is enriched when it's interwoven with diverse perspectives. Sharing stories, listening to others' journeys, and finding commonalities and differences add depth to our understanding. These shared reflections, conversations, and insights form a collective reservoir of wisdom, a treasure trove for generations to come.

In concluding "The Art of Living: Skills for Navigating Life's Ups and Downs," it becomes evident that life isn't about a destination. It's a continuous journey of learning, evolving, and growing. And as we traverse this journey, armed with the skills and insights garnered over time, we realize that the true art of living lies in the ability to draw meaning, joy, and wisdom from each step, making the voyage as enriching as the eventual horizon.

Thus, as we close this chapter, we don't bid farewell. Instead, we invite each reader to embark on their reflective journey, to weave their unique tapestry, and to contribute their distinctive hue to the grand mosaic of life.

www.ingramcontent.com/pod-product-compliance
Lightning Source LLC
Chambersburg PA
CBHW051348280526
45784CB00007B/2868